Natural Grain Free Recipes

Live A Better Life with Grain Free Recipes

BY

Stephanie Sharp

License Notes

Table of Contents

Introduction

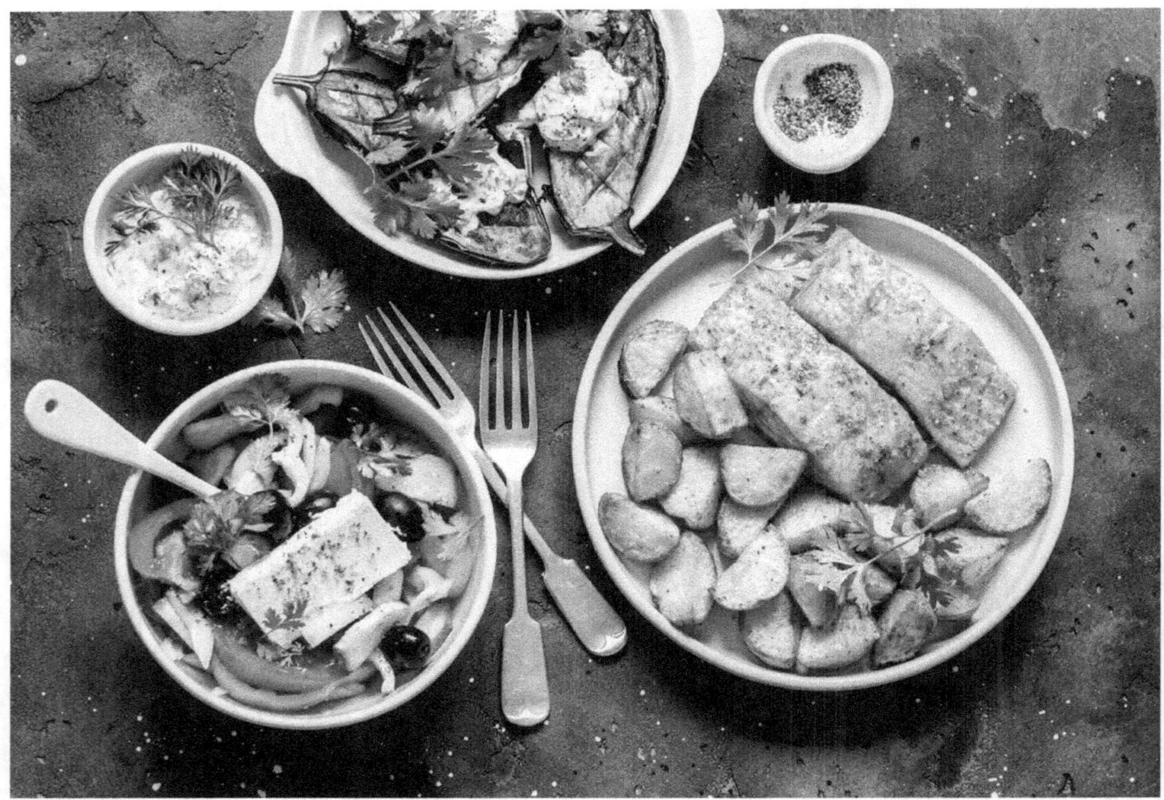

If you look at most people's food choices around the world, you will see many junk food, grains, and artificial flavorings. Many times people start on a diet and then no longer cannot follow it through because they cannot control their cravings. A natural diet can leave you with many healthy food options. You will not run out of food options because you can have everything that is grain free. Modern chefs have invented many items that can substitute grains too. If you really crave for a cake, bread, or crispy coated snacks, you can use grain free flour like coconut flour, almond flour, and for rice you can make cauliflower rice, etc. If you crave for noodles, you can enjoy zucchini noodles, carrot noodles, zicama noodles, or you can make noodles using almond flour too at home.

With the need of modern time, there are available grain free noodles, rice, tortillas in most supermarkets. In this book, you will find 30 delicious grain free natural recipes that are very easy to cook. Feel free to cook them and live a healthier life.

Simple Fruit Salad

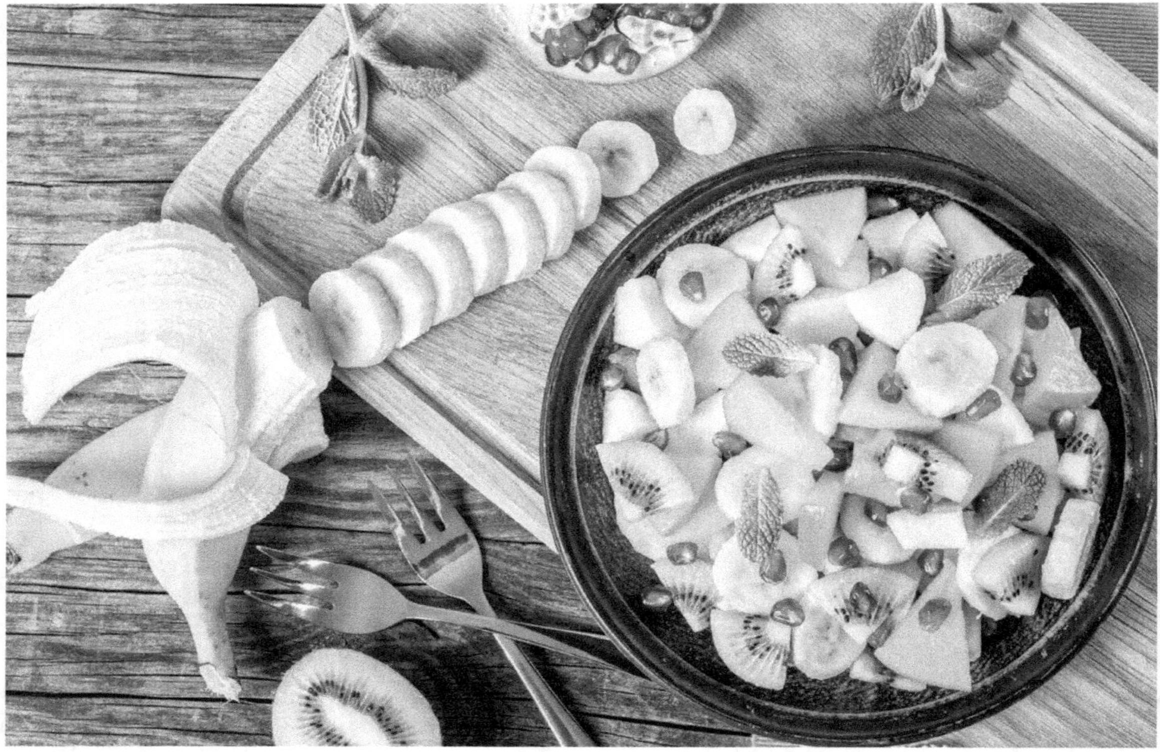

This is a very simple fruit salad which has superfood like apple, kiwi and banana. I have used grapes, tangerines and mangoes. This is heaven in a bowl for any fruit lover.

Serving size: 4

Cooking Time: -

Ingredients:

- 2 apples, cubed
- 2 tangerines, chopped
- 2 ripe bananas, chopped
- 3 kiwis, chopped
- 1 large mango, diced
- ½ cup grapes, cut in half
- 1 tbsp honey
- A pinch of sea salt
- A pinch of apple cider vinegar

Instructions:

Combine the honey, sea salt and apple cider vinegar. Mix well. Set aside for now.

Combine all the fruits in a salad bowl. Add the honey mix and toss well.

Serve cold.

Vegetarian Curry

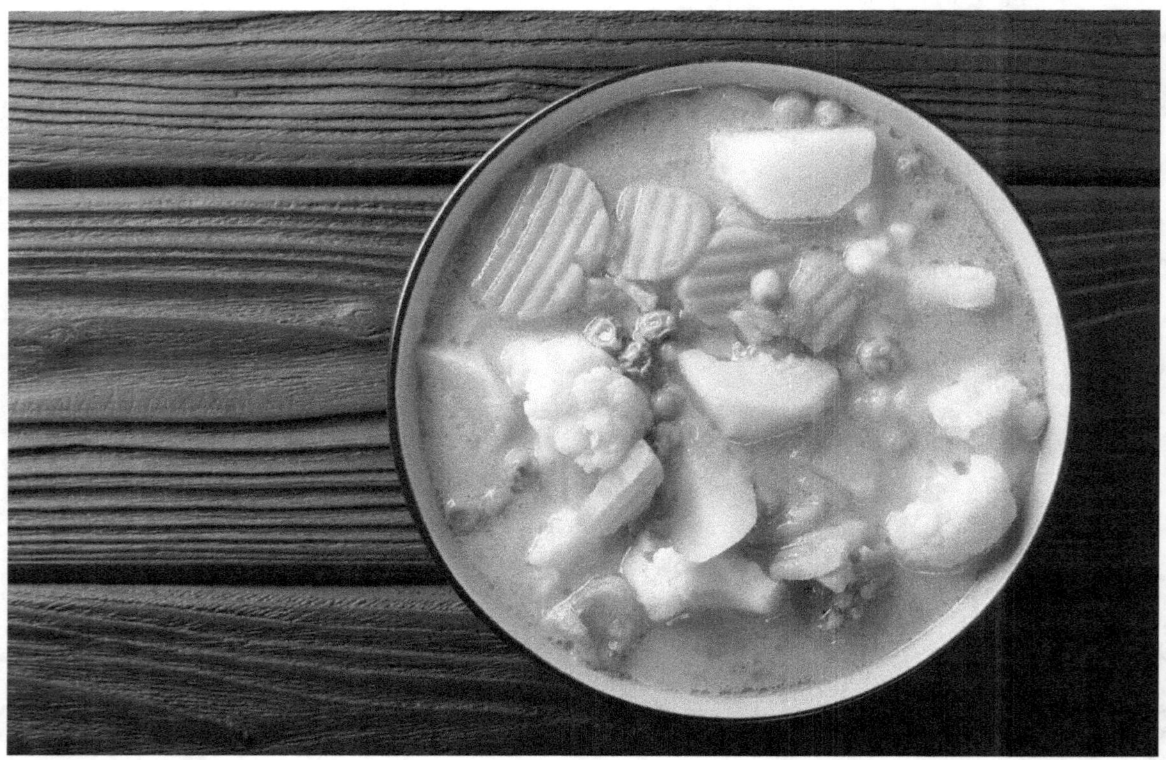

Do you enjoy eating vegetables? If so, you will love this delicious curry with fresh veggies, spices, herbs, and the thick gravy.

Serving size: 4

Cooking Time: 20 Minutes

Ingredients:

- 2 cups vegetable stock
- ½ cup peas
- ½ cup baby malabar spinach
- 1 cup cauliflower florets, diced
- 1 cup sliced carrots
- 2 tomatoes, chopped
- 1 tsp tamarind paste
- 1 cup cubed tofu
- 1 tbsp oil
- Salt to taste
- ½ tsp turmeric
- 1 tsp cumin
- 1 tsp red chili powder
- 1 tsp ginger paste
- 1 tsp garlic paste
- 2 onions, sliced
- 1 green chili

Instructions:

In your large wok, add the oil and fry the onion slices for 1 minute.

Add the ginger and garlic paste. Add ½ cup of vegetable stock.

Add the dry spices and cook for 5 minutes.

Add the cauliflower, carrot, tofu and cook for 5 minutes.

Add the tomatoes, vegetable stock, green chili, spinach, tamarind paste and peas.

Cover and cook on high heat for 10 minutes.

Serve hot.

Grilled Zucchini with Cheese and Pecans

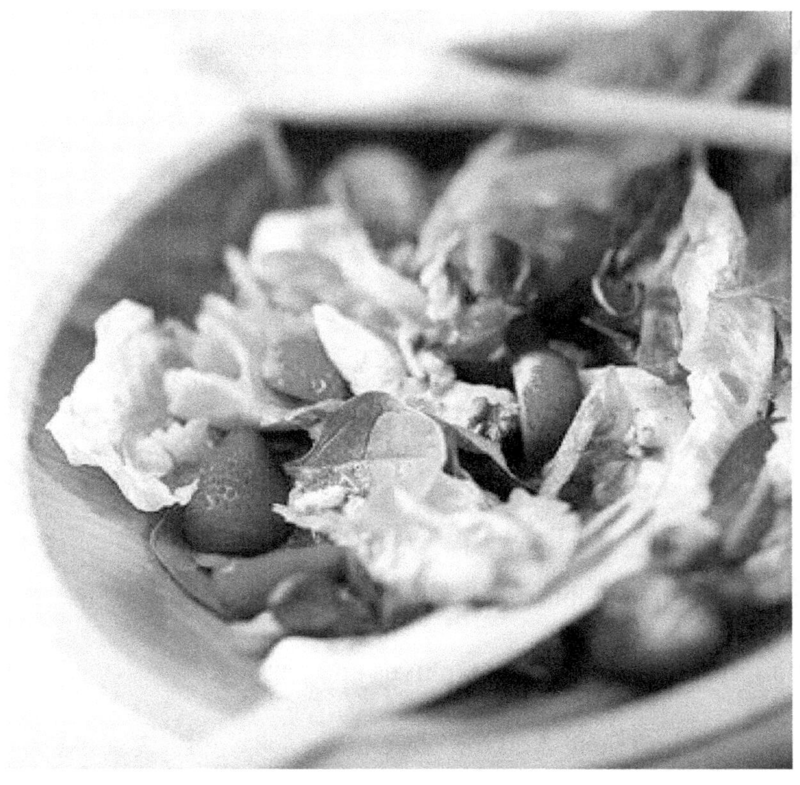

Zucchini slices are grilled and topped with thinly sliced cheese and toasted pecans. Then, herbs are added to enhance the flavors.

Serving size: 4

Cooking Time: 10 Minutes

Ingredients:

- 2 cups zucchini
- 1 cup thinly sliced cheddar cheese
- 4 tbsp pecans, toasted
- Salt and pepper to taste
- 1 tbsp olive oil
- ¼ tsp cumin
- 2 tbsp curry leaves
- Fresh chives, chopped
- Fresh parsley, chopped

Instructions:

Cut off the zucchini stem and cut it into ½ inch slices.

Coat the zucchini in salt, pepper, cumin, chives and parsley.

Heat the grill over medium heat. Add the olive oil.

Grill the zucchini slices for 3 minutes from both sides.

Arrange on a serving plate.

Add the cheddar cheese slices and toasted pecans on top.

Add the curry leaves on top.

Grilled Fish Flakes with Tomatoes

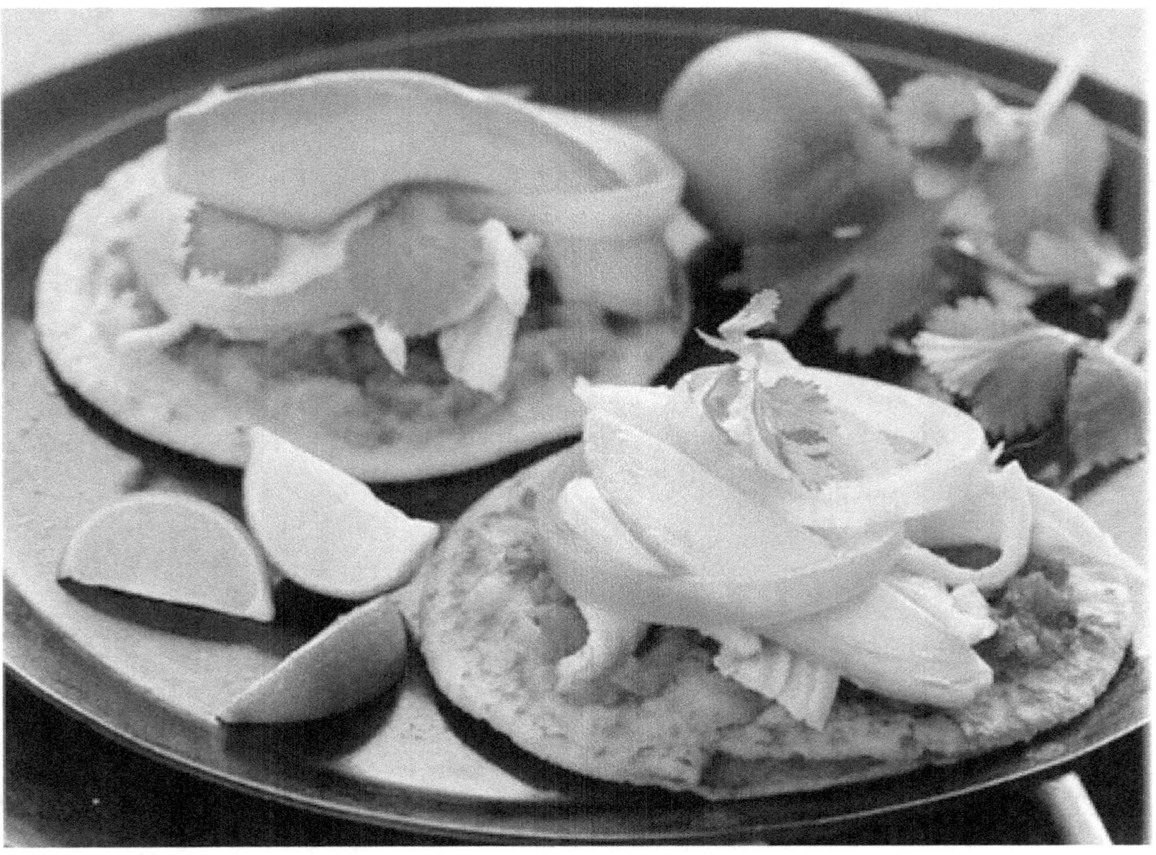

Tuna is pan-fried and then flakes using a fork. Then, it is added with a delicious but simple tomatoes, jalapenos and olive oil salad. The pesto on top adds a lot of flavors.

Serving size: 2

Cooking Time: 15 Minutes

Ingredients:

- 2 tuna fillets
- Salt and pepper to taste
- 1 tbsp soy sauce
- 2 tbsp olive oil
- 1.5 cups cherry tomatoes
- 2 tbsp tomato sauce
- 2 red jalapenos, sliced
- 1 green chili
- 4 tbsp coriander leaves, chopped
- 2 tbsp mint, chopped

Instructions:

Combine the mint, coriander, green chili, 1 tsp olive oil and some salt.

Blend until smooth. Set aside for now.

In a grilling pan, add some oil and add the tuna fillets.

Cook for 4 minutes on each side. Sprinkle some salt and pepper.

Transfer to a plate. Use a fork to flake the fish fillets.

In the grilling pan add some more oil. Add the tomatoes.

Grill for 5 minutes. Transfer to a bowl. Add the jalapeno, tomato sauce, soy sauce and the remaining oil.

Mix well. Add the tuna flakes on top. Add the green chili mix on top.

Avocado Green tomato Brussels Sprouts Salad

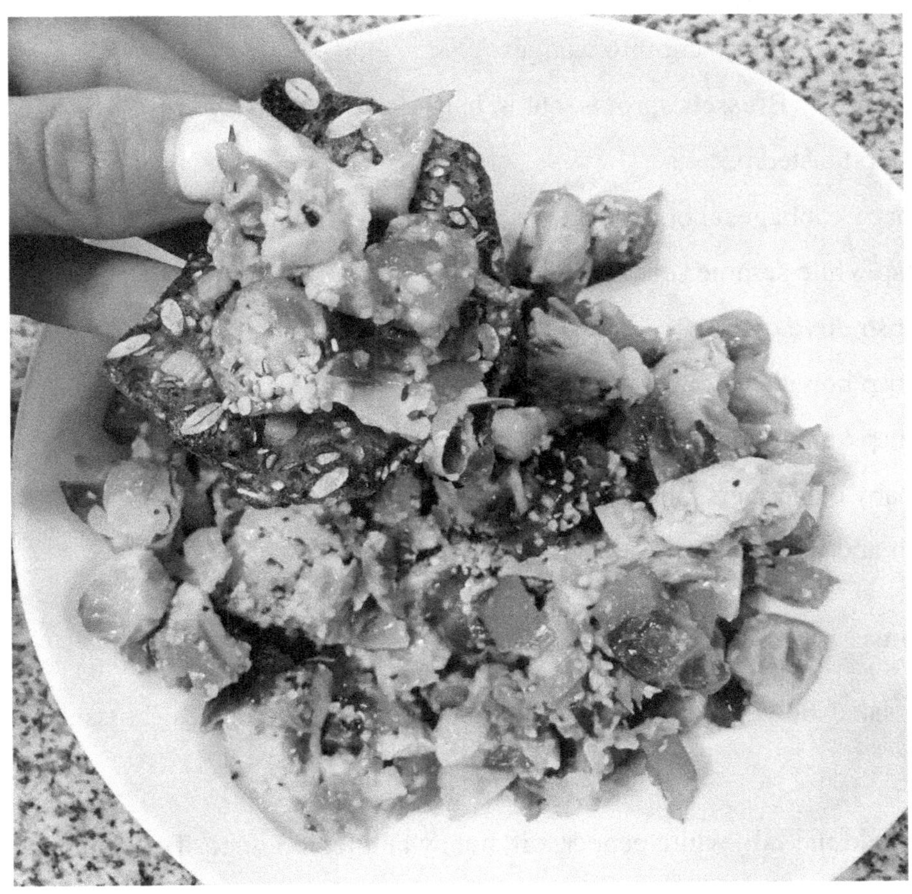

If you are up for a green salad that would definitely cleanse your stomach and body, then this is the quickest remedy for you.

Serving size: 3

Cooking Time: -

Ingredients:

- 2 semi ripe avocados, cut into thick cubes
- 4 green tomatoes, cut into wedges
- 1 cup baby Brussels sprouts, cut in half
- 2 tbsp toasted pecans
- 1 baby cabbage, chopped
- 1 tsp white sesame seeds
- 1 tbsp olive oil
- 1 tbsp honey
- 1 tbsp lemon juice
- 2 baby cucumbers, sliced
- Salt and white pepper to taste

Instructions:

In a large salad bowl, combine the cucumber, avocado, tomatoes, brussels sprouts and cabbage.

Toss well. Add the salt, white pepper, oil, honey and lemon juice. Toss to coat well.

Add the sesame seeds on top and serve.

Chicken Carrot Cheesy Soup

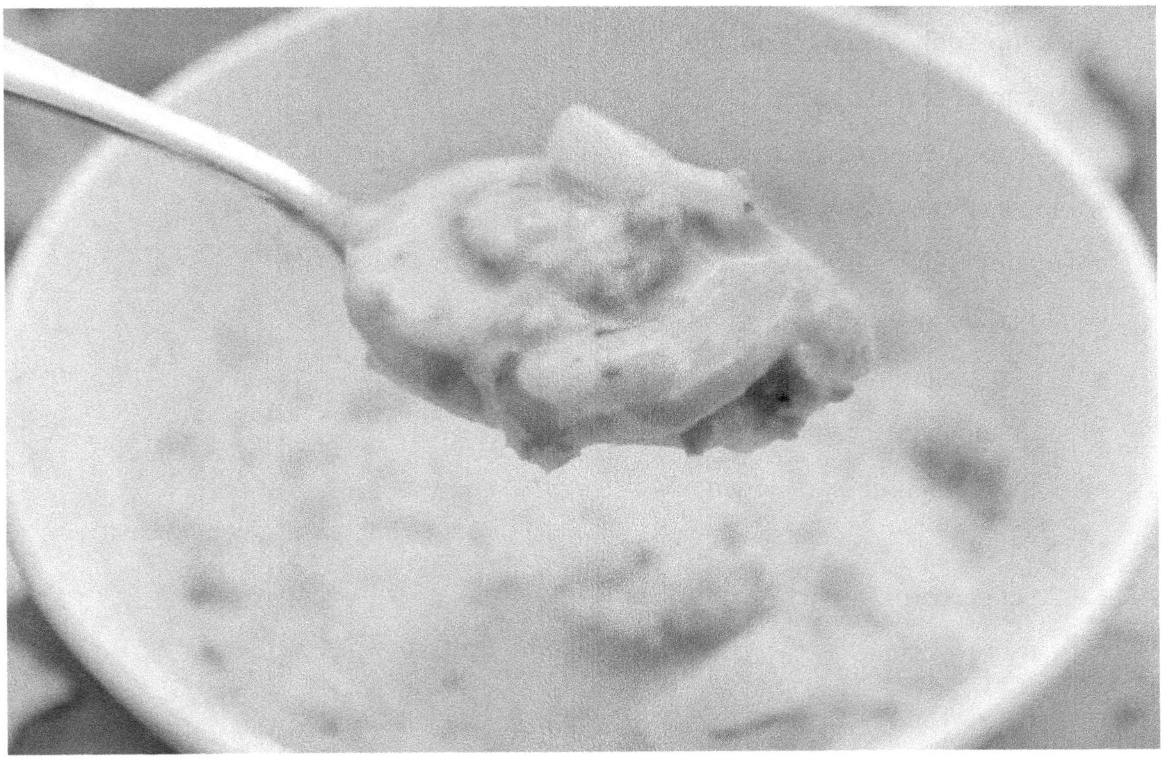

This is a classic clear chicken soup with lots of good vegetables like carrots and cabbage. The cheese in the soup adds a bit of fat which is essential for our body.

Serving size: 4

Cooking Time: 30 Minutes

Ingredients:

- 2 chicken breasts
- 1 cup thinly sliced cheddar cheese
- 1 cup carrot, chopped
- ½ cup shredded cabbage
- Fresh chives, chopped
- 6 cups chicken broth
- 2 garlic cloves, minced
- ½ tsp ginger, minced
- Salt and pepper to taste
- 2 tbsp lemongrass, chopped
- 1 tsp oil
- 2 peppercorns
- 1 tbsp soy sauce

Instructions:

In a pot, add the chicken breasts with the broth.

Add the peppercorn, lemongrass, ginger and garlic.

Cook for 20 minutes. Shred the chicken pieces using a fork. Return it to the pot again.

Add the soy sauce, oil, salt, pepper, carrot, cabbage and chives.

Cook for 10 minutes. Serve hot.

Grilled Fish with Asparagus

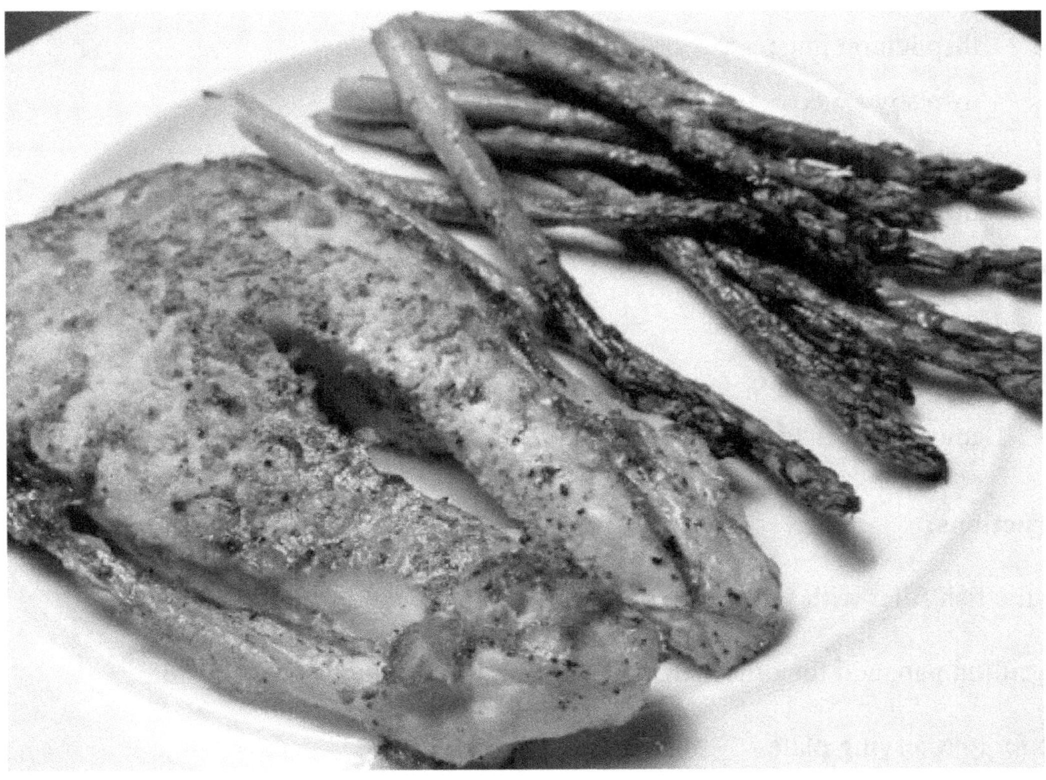

This is a simple fish and asparagus recipe that takes about 10 minutes to make. No time for marinating but it still tastes very delicious.

Serving size: 2

Cooking Time: 10 Minutes

Ingredients:

- 2 cod fillets
- 1 tbsp lemon juice
- 1 tbsp soy sauce
- ½ tsp garlic powder
- Salt and black pepper to taste
- 1 cup asparagus
- 1 tbsp butter
- ½ tsp dried oregano
- Lemon wedges to serve

Instructions:

Coat the fish fillet with salt, garlic powder, oregano and pepper.

In a grilling pan, add the oil. Then, grill the fish for 3 minutes on each side.

Transfer to a serving plate.

In a pan, add the butter. Add the asparagus and sprinkle some salt and oregano.

Toss for 3 minutes. Serve with lemon juice and lemon wedges.

Pan-Fried Fish with Bell Pepper

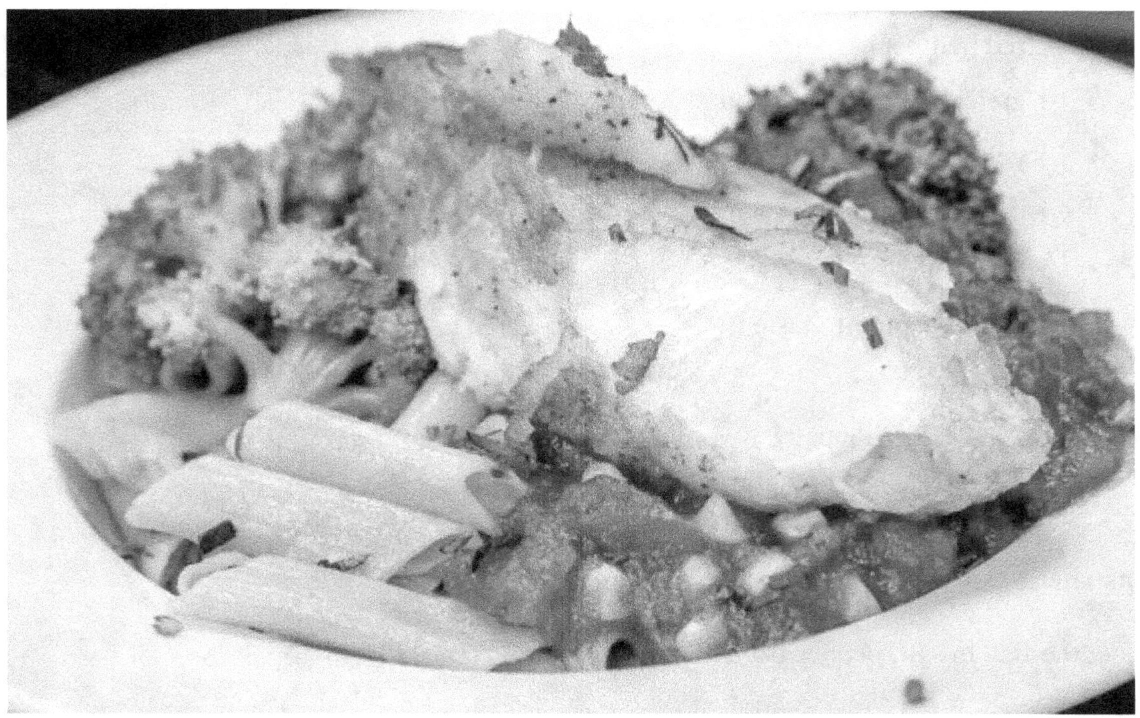

This pan-fried fish tastes so good that you will fall in love with this simple fish recipe. The salad on the side is also very refreshing and quick.'

Serving size: 2

Cooking Time: 10 Minutes

Ingredients:

- 2 cod fillets, boneless, cut into medium chunks
- 1 red bell pepper, diced
- 1 green bell pepper, diced
- 1 yellow bell pepper, diced
- 1 tbsp lemon juice
- 1 tbsp honey
- Salt and pepper to taste
- 1 tbsp butter
- Fresh basil, chopped
- Lime wedges, to serve

Instructions:

Coat the fish in salt, pepper from all sides.

In a pan, add the butter. Add the fish, then cook for 4 minutes or until they become golden in both sides.

Transfer to a serving plate.

In a bowl, combine the bell peppers, basil, salt, pepper, honey and lemon juice. Then, mix well.

Serve with lime wedges on top.

Veggies in Coconut Curry

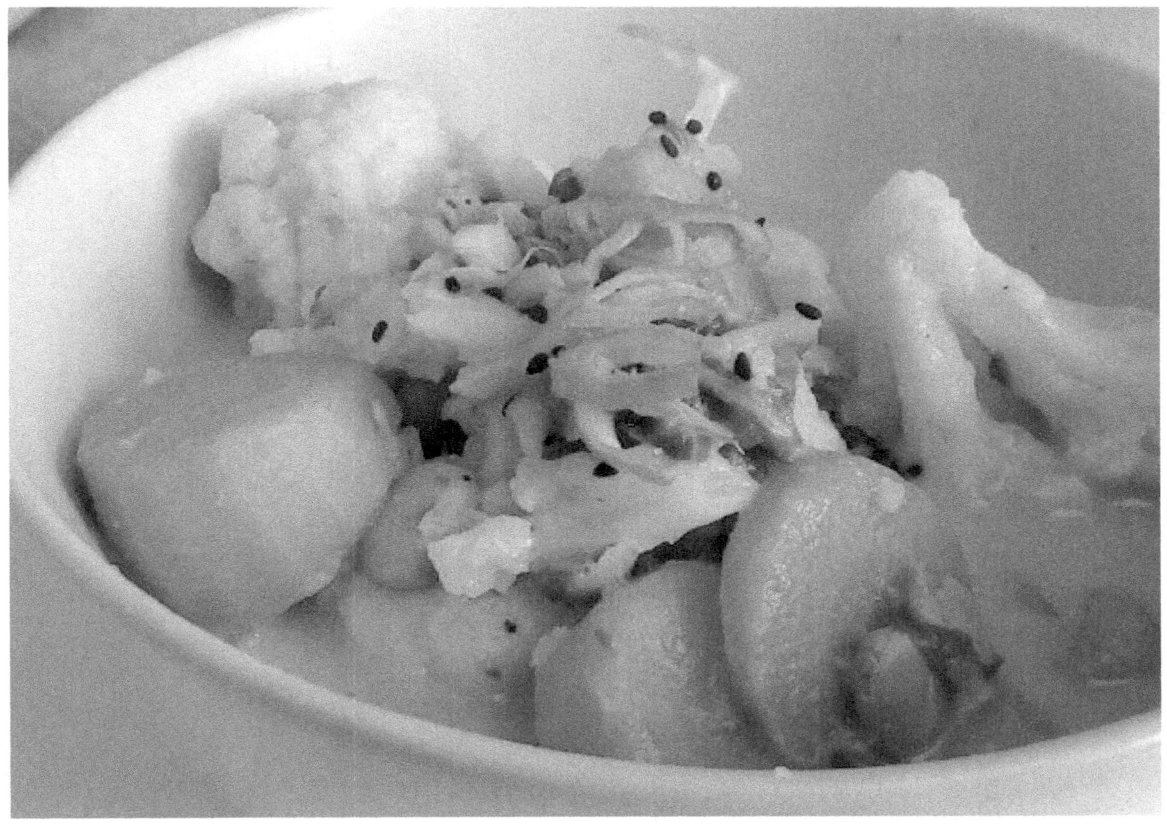

This is a thick gravy curry with carrot, potatoes and lima beans. The parsley in the curry is great too. The coconut milk adds to the flavoring.

Serving size: 4

Cooking Time: 20 Minutes

Ingredients:

- 1 cup boiled lima beans
- 2 cups coconut milk
- 1 cup vegetable stock
- 1 cup cubed potatoes
- 1 cup cubed pumpkin
- 1 cup cubed carrots
- Salt to taste
- 1/3 tsp turmeric
- 1 tsp cumin
- 1 tbsp oil
- Fresh parsley, chopped

Instructions:

In a pressure cooker, add the lima beans and vegetable stock.

Cover and cook for 8 minutes.

Add all the veggies, turmeric, cumin, salt, oil and coconut milk.

Cook for 12 minutes. Add the parsley on top and serve hot.

Beef and Broccoli

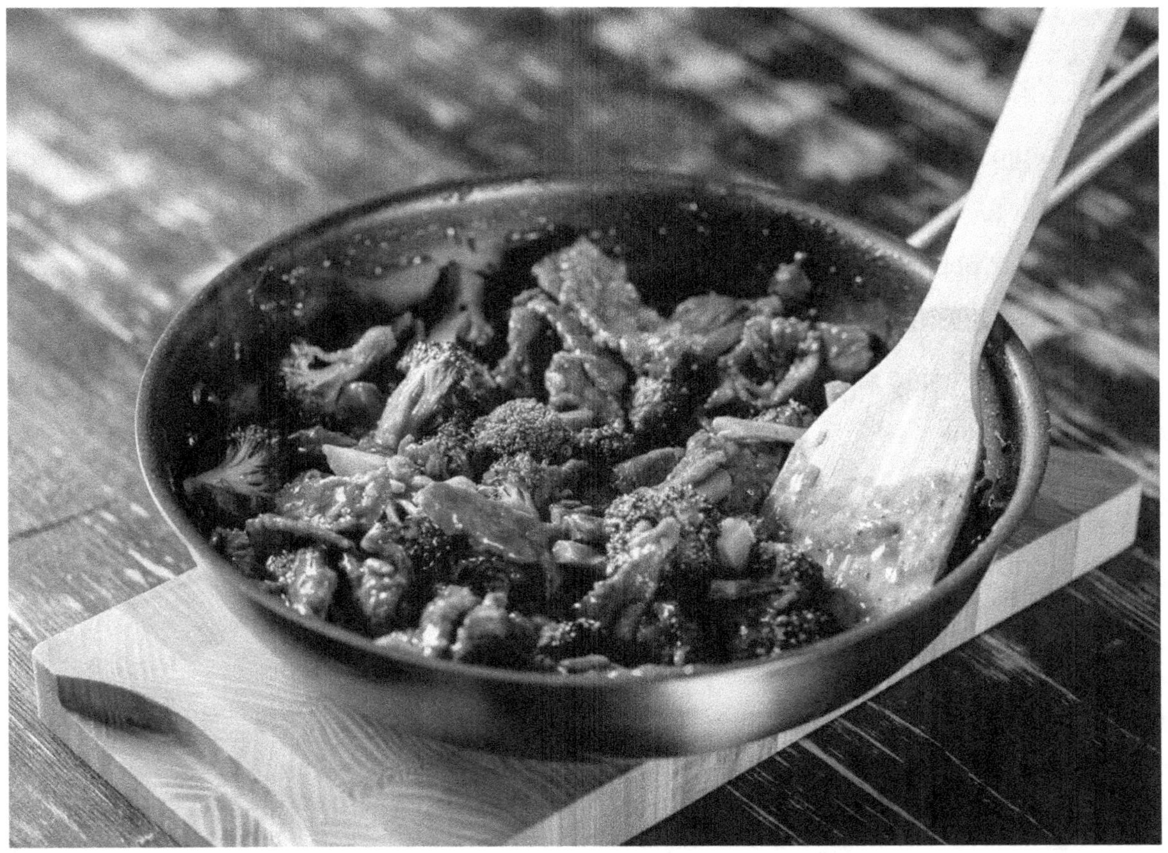

Beef and Broccoli in soy sauce is a combination that is bound to work for any type of audience. You should love it as the flavor is very intense.

Serving size: 4

Cooking Time: 25 Minutes

Ingredients:

- 2 cups beef, boneless, fatless, cut into julienne
- 2 cups broccoli florets, diced
- 4 tbsp soy sauce
- 1 cup beef broth
- Salt to taste
- Black pepper to taste
- 1 tsp chili flakes
- 2 tbsp tomato puree
- 2 tbsp oil
- ¼ tsp cinnamon powder

Instructions:

In a large wok, add the oil.

Toss the beef until it becomes slightly brown.

Add the soy sauce, tomato puree, salt, pepper, cinnamon powder and beef broth.

Cook on high heat for 10 minutes. Add the broccoli and chili flakes.

Cook for 10 minutes. Check the seasoning.

Take off the heat and serve hot.

Creamy Tomato Soup

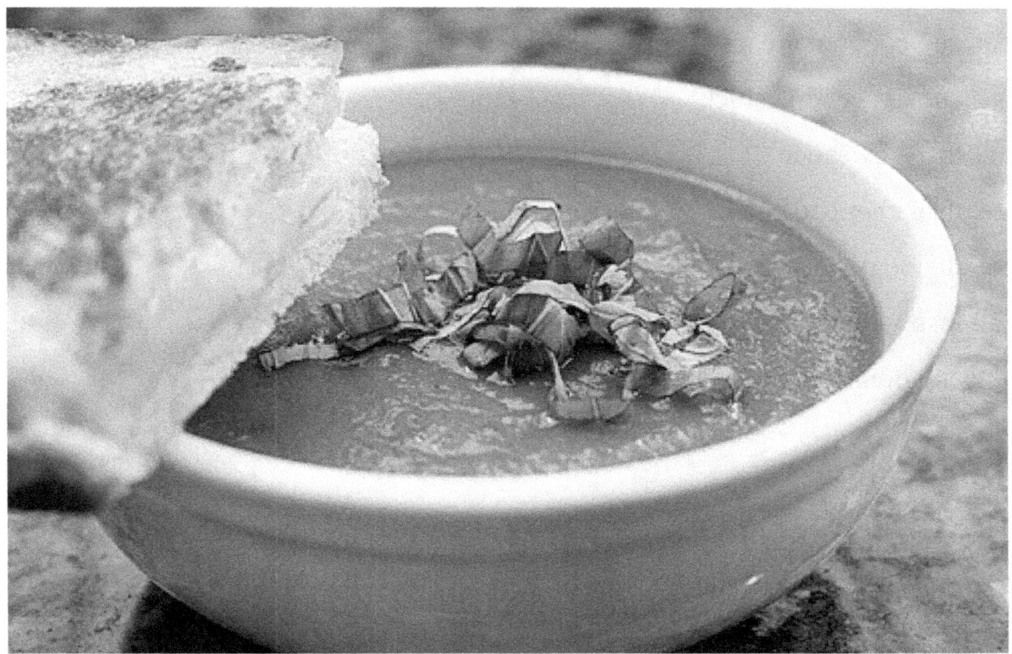

Tomato is very good for our health. Basil also contains many health benefits and coconut cream is very light in texture and has a good flavor. All the ingredients go really well in terms of flavors.

Serving size: 4

Cooking Time: 20 Minutes

Ingredients:

- 2 cups tomato puree
- 1 cup coconut cream
- 2 cups vegetable stock
- 1 tbsp soy sauce
- 2 tbsp chopped basil
- Salt and pepper to taste
- 2 tbsp vinegar
- ½ tsp oregano

Instructions:

In a pot, combine the tomato puree with the vegetable stock.

Add the basil, soy sauce, salt, pepper, oregano and vinegar. Then, cook for 15 minutes.

Add the coconut cream and cook for 5 minutes.

Use an electric hand blender to blend the mixture into a smooth paste.

Serve hot.

Thick Broccoli Carrot Soup

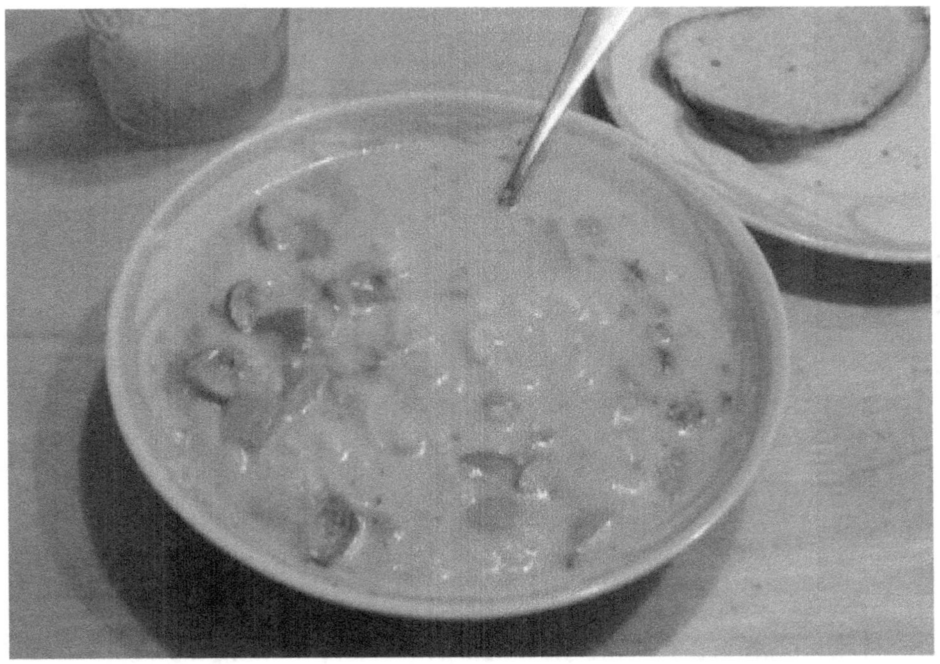

When you are bored with the clear soups, it is time to add some thickness to it by pouring in some heavy cream, coconut milk and delicious spices.

Serving size: 4

Cooking Time: 20 Minutes

Ingredients:

- 1 cup broccoli with stem, chopped
- 1 cup carrot, grated
- 1 green chili, deseeded, chopped
- Fresh parsley, chopped
- Salt to taste
- 2 tbsp celery, chopped
- 2 cup heavy cream
- 1 cup vegetable stock
- 2 tbsp lemongrass, chopped
- ¼ tsp paprika

Instructions:

In your large pot, combine the vegetable stock with celery, lemongrass, carrot and broccoli.

Cook for 10 minutes. Add the heavy cream, green chili, parsley, paprika and salt. Then, cook for 10 minutes.

Serve hot.

Spicy Crab Salad

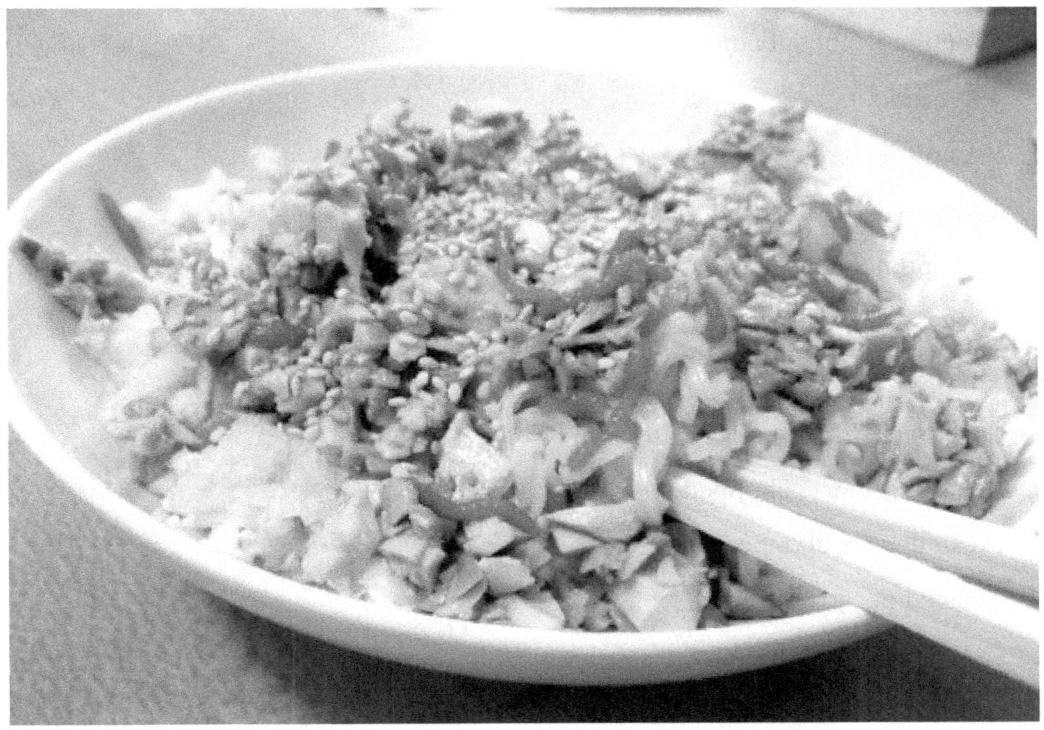

If you want to enjoy a good homemade but yet restaurant quality crab salad, try this recipe. The ingredients are simple but very healthy and refreshing.

Serving size: 2

Cooking Time: 10 Minutes

Ingredients:

- 1 cup crab meat
- ½ cup red cabbage, diced
- 1 avocado, cubed
- ½ cup spinach, chopped
- 1 yellow bell pepper, chopped
- Salt and pepper to taste
- 1 tbsp lemon juice
- 1 tbsp honey
- 1 tsp butter
- Fresh rosemary, chopped
- Fresh thyme, chopped
- Toasted pecans to serve

Instructions:

In your skillet, melt the butter and fry the crab for 3 minutes. Sprinkle some salt and pepper on top.

Transfer to a salad bowl.

Add the cabbage, spinach, bell pepper, rosemary and thyme. Then, mix well.

Add the lemon juice and honey, and sprinkle some more salt and pepper.

Toss well. Add the toasted pecans on top and serve.

Baby Potatoes Green Beans in Pesto

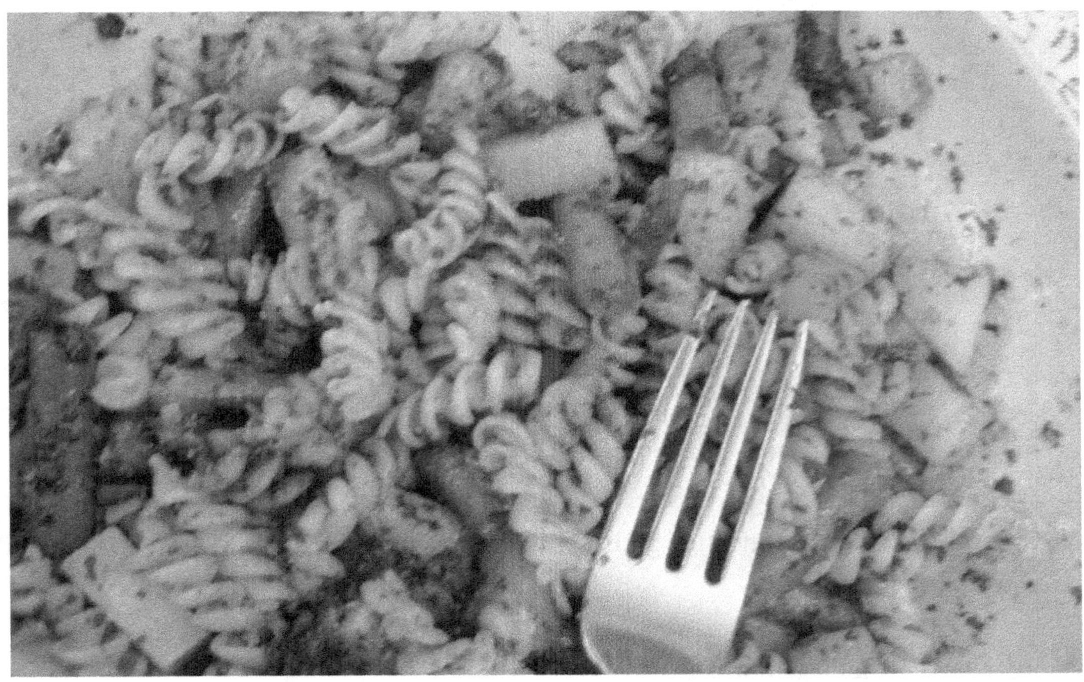

Baby potatoes taste really good in a pesto sauce. Adding green beans complements the baby potatoes well. It looks very refreshing to combine yellowish and green color in the plate.

Serving size: 4

Cooking Time: 15 Minutes

Ingredients:

- 2 cups baby potatoes
- 1.5 cups green beans cut in half
- 2 green chilies
- ½ cup coriander leaves
- 2 tbsp basil leaves
- 1 tbsp mint leaves
- Salt and pepper to taste
- 2 tbsp butter

Instructions:

In a food processor, combine the green chilies, coriander, mint and basil. Blend until smooth.

In a nonstick pan, melt the butter.

Add the baby potatoes. Cover with lid. Cook until they get a golden color.

Add the green beans. Sprinkle the salt and pepper.

Add the pesto sauce and stir for 8 minutes on medium low heat.

Serve hot.

Beef Steak with Garlic Tomato Sauce

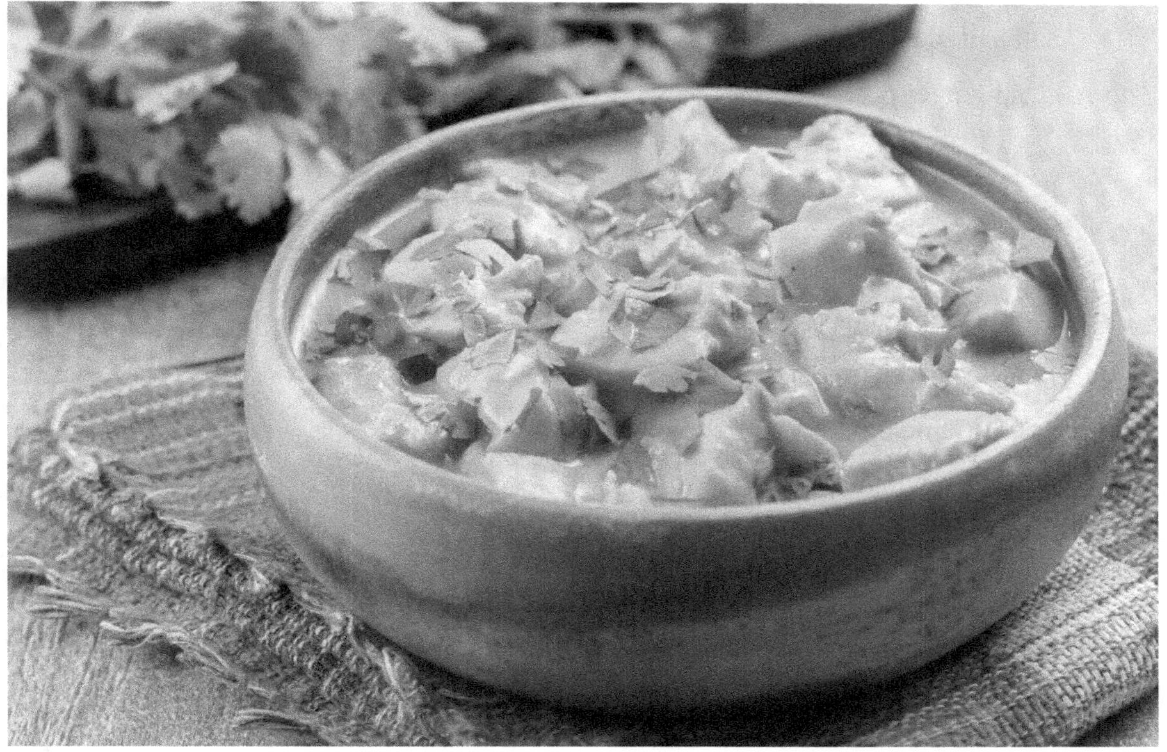

Beef steak is very versatile recipe and anyone can make marinate sauces of his/her choice to make it unique. It is usually kept simple because when you cook the beef on the grill or bake it, it contains a distinct flavor of its own; so you do not need too many ingredients to make it extra special. This recipe however is served with a delicious garlic and tomato sauce.

Serving size: 2

Cooking Time: 15 Minutes

Ingredients:

- 2 beef steak
- Salt and black pepper to taste
- ¼ tsp ginger powder
- ¼ tsp garlic powder
- 1 tbsp butter
- 2 tbsp butter
- 2 tomatoes, chopped
- 4 garlic cloves, minced
- 1 tsp sesame oil
- ½ cup arugula leaves, to serve

Instructions:

Marinate the beef steaks with garlic powder, ginger powder, salt and pepper, and let it sit for 2 hours.

In a grill, add the butter and grill the beef for 5 minutes on each side.

Let it rest for some time. Meanwhile, make the sauce.

In a pan, add the sesame oil.

Add the garlic. Then, cook for 1 minute.

Next, add the tomatoes, and some salt and pepper.

Toss for 3 minutes. Serve the steam on top of the arugula leaves. Top with the garlic sauce.

Onion Caramelized Cod with Veggies

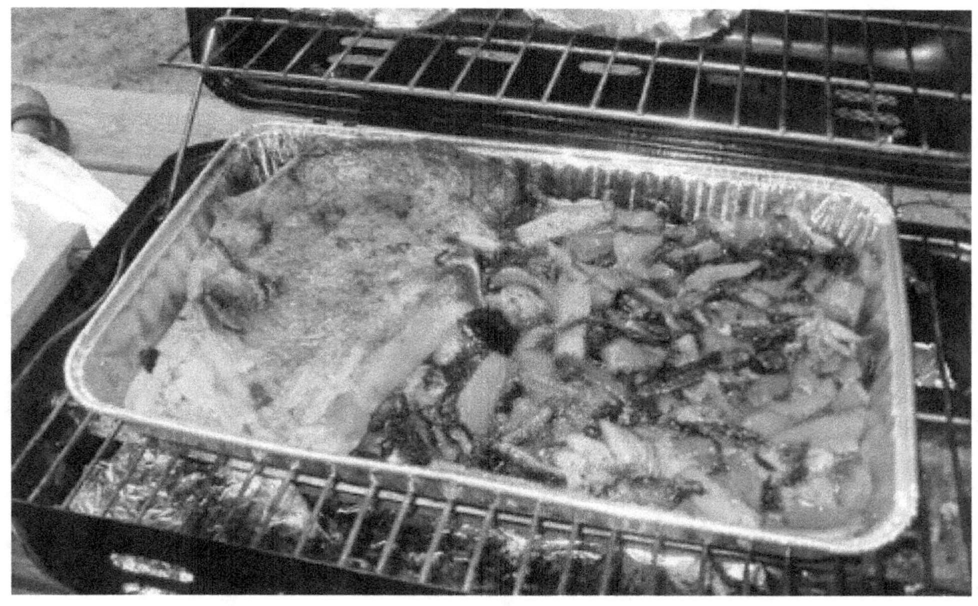

If you have not tried caramelized fish before, try this. You will be amazed. You can try it with any fish of your choice. I have used baby edamame, broccoli and bell pepper for veggies. You can use veggies you like.

Serving size: 2

Cooking Time: 15 Minutes

Ingredients:

- 2 cod fillets
- 1 cup sliced onion
- ½ cup broccoli, diced
- ½ cup baby edamame
- 1 red bell pepper, sliced
- Salt and pepper to taste
- 1 tbsp soy sauce
- 1 tbsp oil
- 1 tbsp butter
- ¼ tsp dried oregano

Instructions:

In your pan, heat the oil and add the onion.

Cook until they become caramelized.

Add the cod fillets on top of the caramelized onions.

Sprinkle some salt and pepper and add some soy sauce.

Cook for 3 minutes on each side, and make sure the onions do not get burnt.

Transfer them onto your serving plate.

In another skillet, melt the butter.

Add the broccoli and baby edamame and toss for 3 minutes.

Add the bell pepper, oregano, and salt and pepper.

Cook for another 3 minutes. Serve with the fish.

Chicken Drumstick and Veggie Stir-Fry

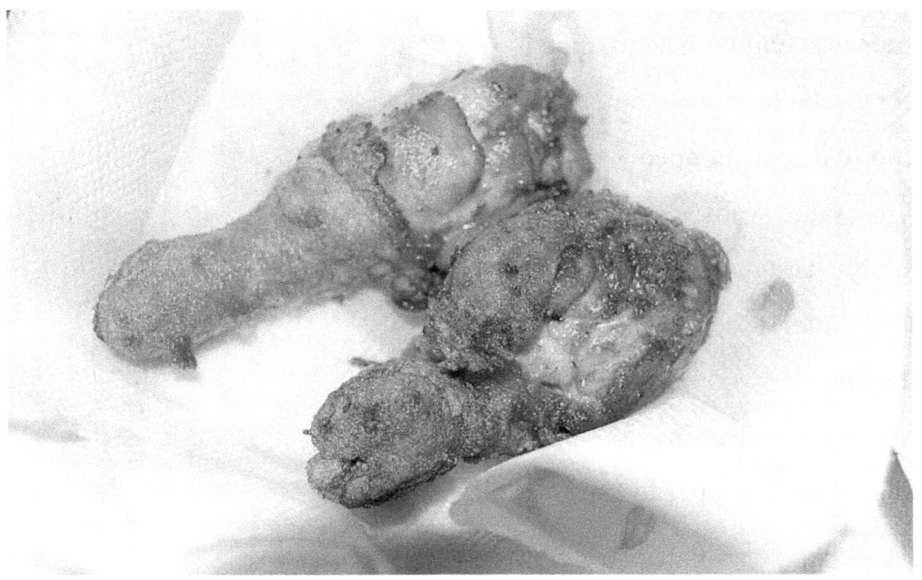

Stir-fry is quick and easy but to twist things up, try this recipe. It is a unique stir-fry dish with chicken drumsticks in it. It looks fabulous and tastes even better.

Serving size: 6

Cooking Time: 25 Minutes

Ingredients:

- 8 chicken drumsticks
- 2 cups broccoli with stem, diced
- 2 cups cubed carrot
- 1 cup scallion, chopped
- 2 tsp sesame seeds
- 2 cups asparagus, cut in half
- 2 tbsp butter
- 2 tbsp soy sauce
- 2 tbsp apple cider vinegar
- Salt and black pepper to taste
- 2 red jalapeno pepper, chopped
- Fresh thyme, chopped
- 2 onions, sliced
- 4 garlic cloves, minced
- 1 tbsp honey
- 2 tbsp curry leaves
- 2 red bell pepper, chopped

Instructions:

Coat the chicken drumsticks in honey, 1 tsp soy sauce, salt and pepper.

In a large wok, melt the butter. Fry the chicken until it becomes golden in color.

Transfer the chicken onto a plate.

In the same wok, add the garlic, onion, and cook for 1 minute.

Add the broccoli with stem. Add the carrots. Cook for 4 minutes.

Add the asparagus, bell pepper, jalapeno pepper and curry leaves.

Cook for 3 minutes. Add the salt, pepper, soy sauce, apple cider vinegar, thyme and scallion, and cook for 8 minutes.

Add the sesame seeds and return the chicken in the wok.

Toss for 5 minutes. Serve hot.

Tofu Carrot Green Bean Stir-Fry

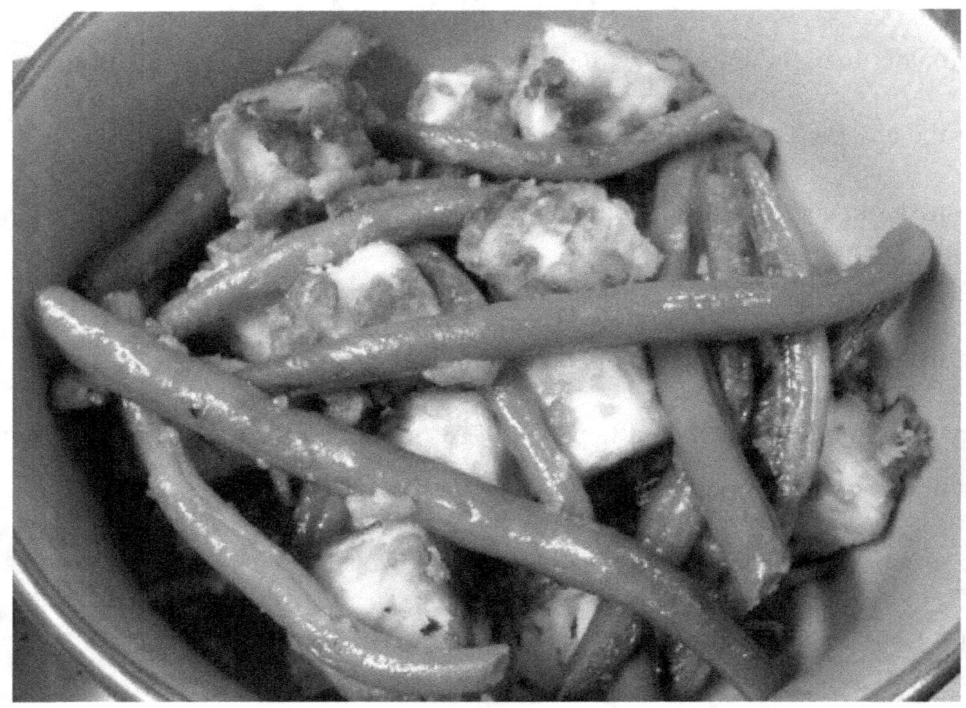

This is a delicious vegan stir-fry recipe which even people who are not vegan would love.

Serving size: 4

Cooking Time: 15 Minutes

Ingredients:

- 2 cups extra firm tofu
- 1.5 cups carrot, cut into thick 2 inch slices
- 1.5 cups green beans, cut in half
- 2 garlic cloves, sliced
- 1 inch ginger, sliced
- 2 tbsp soy sauce
- Salt to taste
- Black pepper to taste
- 2 tbsp butter

Instructions:

In a skillet, melt the butter.

Add the tofu and fry for 4 minutes or until they become golden.

Transfer the tofu on a kitchen paper.

In the same skillet, fry the ginger and garlic.

Add the carrots and toss for 3 minutes.

Add the green beans and toss for 2 minutes.

Return the tofu and add the soy sauce and salt, pepper. Then, cook for 4 minutes.

Serve hot.

Broccoli Bell Pepper Shrimp Stir-Fry

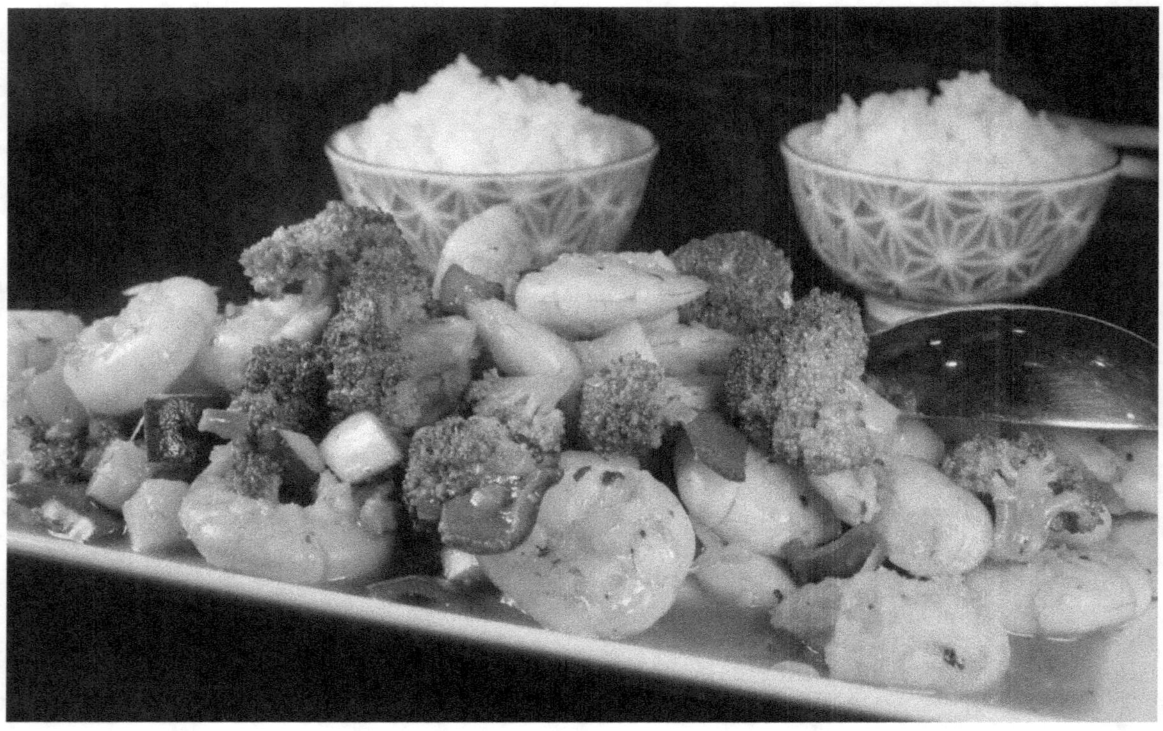

Have you ever tried making stir-fries with shrimp in it? If you haven't, you should try this recipe as it does not require any extra effort or time to make this. The flavors of your stir-fry get enhanced when you add the shrimp.

Serving size: 4

Cooking Time: 15 Minutes

Ingredients:

- 2 cups medium shrimp, cleaned, skin removed
- 2 green bell pepper, julienned
- 1.5 cups broccoli florets, diced
- 2 red bell pepper, julienned
- ½ cup baby snap peas
- 2 tbsp olive oil
- Salt and pepper to taste
- Fresh thyme, chopped
- 2 tbsp soy sauce
- 1/3 tsp dried oregano

Instructions:

In a large pan, heat the oil. Add the shrimp and toss for 2 minutes.

Transfer to a kitchen paper.

In the same pan, add the broccoli and cook for 3 minutes.

Add the snap peas, bell peppers and soy sauce.

Toss for 3 minutes. Return the shrimp in the pan again.

Add the salt, pepper and oregano, and cook for 5 minutes.

Serve with thyme on top.

Cauliflower Broccoli Coconut Curry

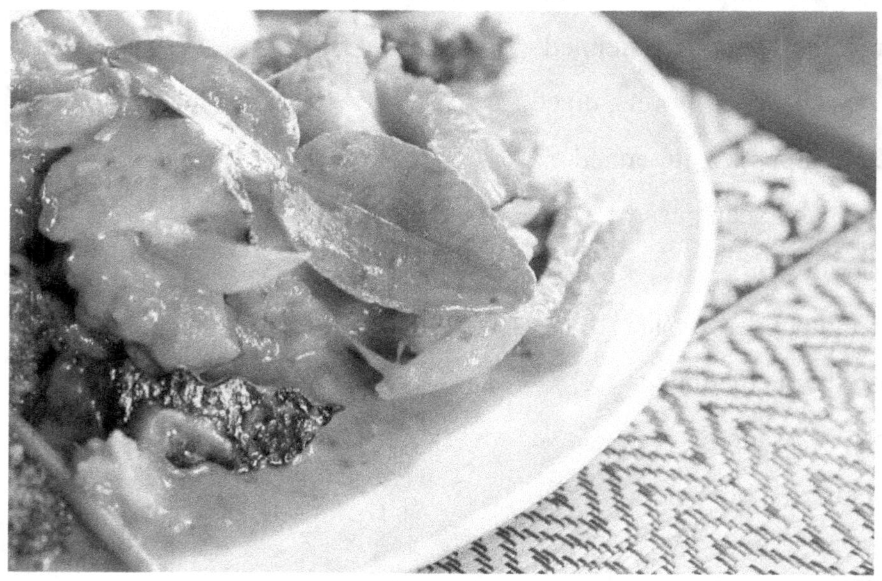

Cauliflower and Broccoli, both are very good for our health. These veggies are kind of similar in terms of texture and they complement each other when used in the same curry. So, this thick coconut curry is dedicated to only broccoli and cauliflower.

Serving size: 4

Cooking Time: 25 Minutes

Ingredients:

- 1.5 cups broccoli florets, diced
- 1.5 cups cauliflower florets, diced
- 1 onion, chopped
- 2 garlic cloves, minced
- 1 tsp minced ginger
- ¼ tsp turmeric
- ¼ tsp cumin
- Salt and white pepper to taste
- 1 tbsp tomato sauce
- 1 tsp sugar
- 2 cups coconut milk
- 1/3 tsp dried oregano
- 2 tbsp butter

Instructions:

In a large pot, melt the butter. Add the broccoli and cauliflower. Then, toss until they get slightly golden.

Transfer to a plate.

Next, in the same pot, add the ginger, garlic and onion.

Toss for 2 minutes. Add the tomato sauce, coconut milk, oregano, salt, cumin, turmeric and pepper, and cook for 5 minutes.

Add the cauliflower and broccoli. Then, cook for 10 minutes.

Serve hot.

Spicy Baked Chicken Drumstick

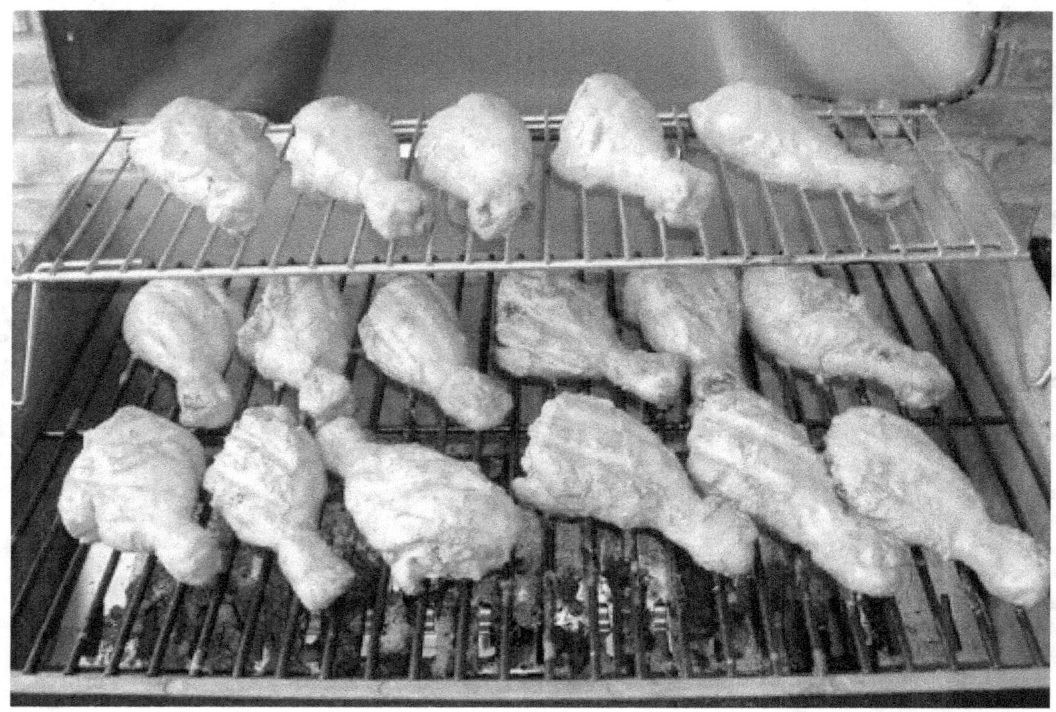

If you are looking for a simply clean appetizer recipe where you do not want to spend too much time in your own kitchen; but you still want crowd pleasing food, this is the recipe you should try.

Serving size: 4

Cooking Time: 35 Minutes

Ingredients:

- 2 lb. chicken drumsticks
- 1 tsp chili flakes
- ½ tsp paprika
- 1 tsp garlic powder
- 1 tsp ginger powder
- 2 tbsp soy sauce
- Salt to taste
- 1 tbsp olive oil

Instructions:

In your bowl, combine the olive oil, salt, paprika, soy sauce, sugar, ginger, garlic and chili flakes.

Mix well and add the drumsticks. Coat well and let them marinate for 2 hours.

Preheat the oven to 380 degrees F.

Add aluminum foil on your baking tray.

Arrange the drumsticks and bake for 20 minutes. Flip them and bake for another 15 minutes.

Serve warm.

Curried Veggies

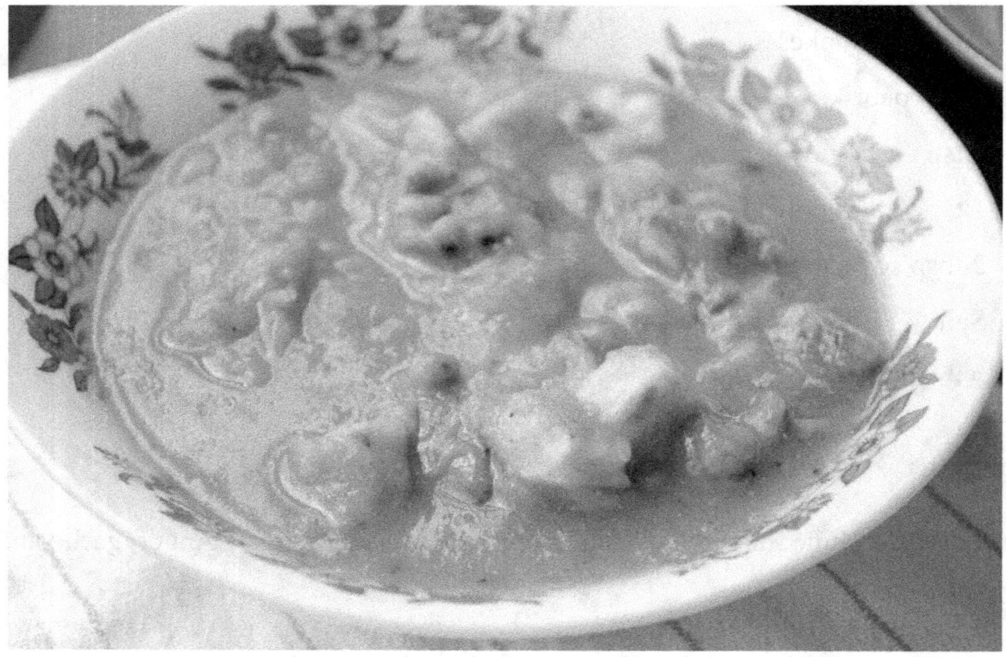

This is a unique vegetarian dish that any vegetarian would love. It contains vegetables like sweet potatoes, carrots and peas. Feel free to add any other veggies.

Serving size: 4

Cooking Time: 20 Minutes

Ingredients:

- 2 cups coconut milk
- 1 cup sweet potato, cubed
- 1 cup carrot, cubed
- 1 cup pea
- Salt and white pepper to taste
- ¼ tsp turmeric
- 1 tsp ginger powder
- 1 tsp garlic powder
- 2 onions, chopped
- 1 cup heavy cream

Instructions:

In a large pot, add the butter.

Add the onion and toss for 1 minute.

Add the cubed sweet potatoes and carrots.

Toss for 2 minutes and add the ginger, garlic, turmeric, salt and pepper, and stir for 5 minutes.

Add the peas and coconut milk and bring it to boil.

Simmer for 5 minutes and add the heavy cream.

Cook for 5 minutes. Serve hot.

Herby Pan Grilled Chicken Breasts

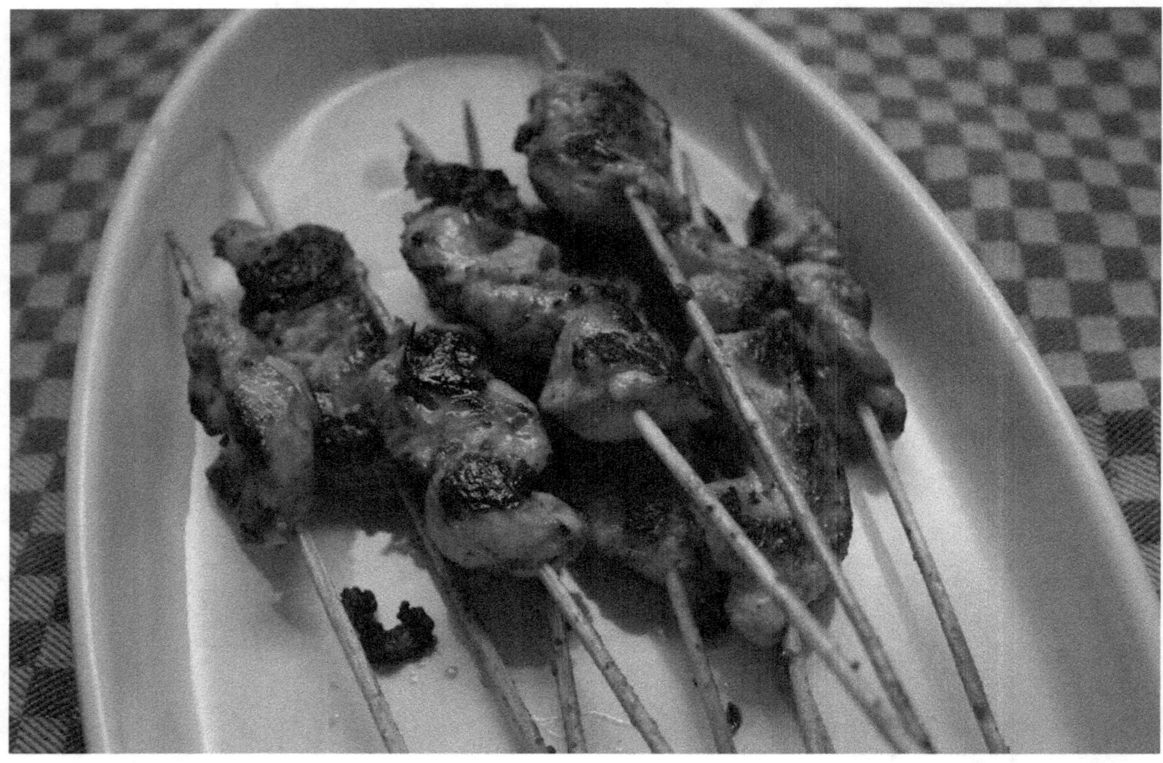

If you are in a nervous hurry, but you want something that is refreshing, high in protein and yet delicious! This is the quickest remedy for you.

Serving size: 4

Cooking Time: 15 Minutes

Ingredients:

- 4 chicken breasts
- 1 tbsp orange juice
- 1 tbsp lemon juice
- 1 tsp chopped chives
- 1 tsp chopped parsley
- Salt and black pepper to taste
- 2 tbsp butter
- Fresh coriander, chopped
- 1 tsp garlic powder

Instructions:

Combine the garlic powder, salt, pepper, parsley, chives, lemon juice and orange juice together.

Coat the chicken breast in it. Let it sit for 10 minutes.

Add butter to your grilling pan.

Grill for 4 minutes on each side.

Add more coriander on top and serve.

Chicken Zucchini Sesame Salad

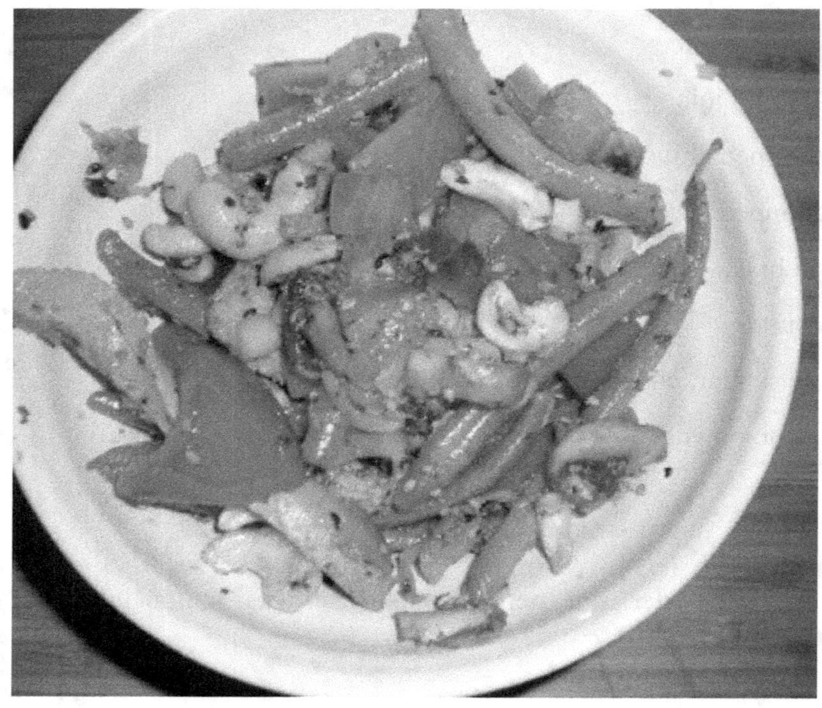

Thinly sliced zucchini is combined with thinly julienned chicken. Then, white sesame seeds and scallions are added on top. This is definitely a delicious and healthy dish you can try within 20 minutes.

Serving size: 4

Cooking Time: 20 Minutes

Ingredients:

- 2 cups zucchini, sliced
- 1 tbsp sesame seeds
- 4 chicken breasts, cut into julienne
- Salt and pepper to taste
- 2 tbsp soy sauce
- 1 onion, chopped
- 2 green chilies, cut in half
- 2 tbsp scallions, chopped
- 2 tbsp butter
- 1 tsp sugar

Instructions:

In a pan, melt the butter and toss the chicken until it gets a golden color.

Add the onion, zucchini and chilies, and toss for 2 minutes.

Add the salt, pepper and soy sauce. Then, cook for 5 minutes.

Add the sugar and toss for 8 minutes.

Add the scallion and sesame seeds on top.

Serve hot.

Chicken Bacon Egg Salad

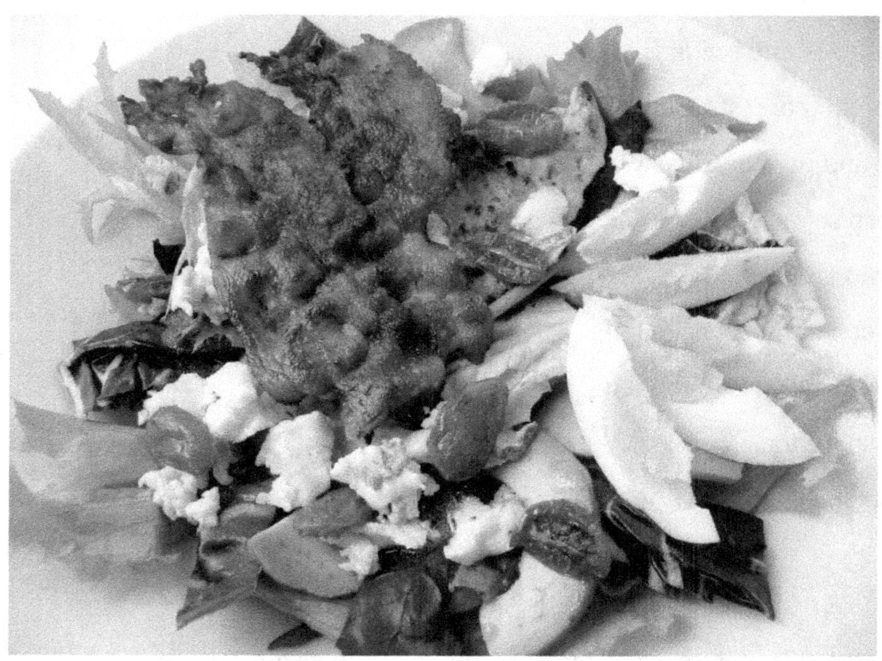

This is a very unique salad with boiled eggs, chicken bacon, black cumin seeds, cherry tomatoes and Napa cabbage.

Serving size: 4

Cooking Time: 15 Minutes

Ingredients:

- 3 eggs
- 2 cups Napa cabbage, chopped
- 1 tsp black cumin seeds
- 1/3 cup chicken bacon bits
- 1 cup cherry tomatoes, cut in half
- 3 tbsp mayo
- 1 tbsp lemon juice
- 1 tbsp honey
- Salt and pepper to taste
- 1 tbsp olive oil

Instructions:

In a nonstick pan, add the oil and fry the chicken bacon for 5 minutes. Transfer to a plate.

In a pot, boil the eggs for 6 minutes. Let them cool down. Remove the shells. Cut them in half.

In a salad bowl, combine the cabbage, cherry tomatoes, black cumin seeds and chicken bacon, and mix well.

Add the salt, pepper, honey, lemon juice and mayo, and mix again.

Add the boiled eggs on top and serve.

Broccoli Tofu Mushroom Bok Choy Stir-Fry

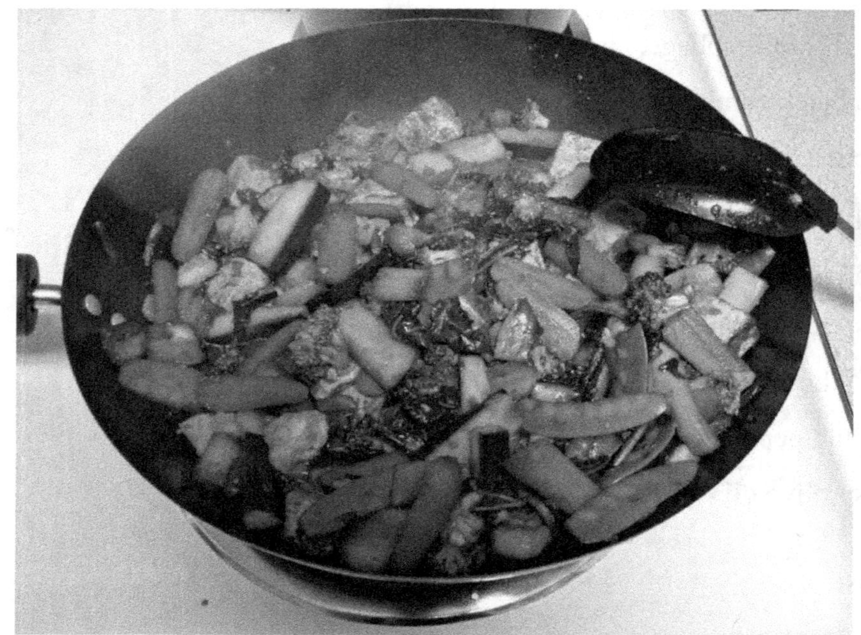

If you are a vegan or a vegetarian, you must love this combination. It contains tofu, mushroom and broccoli. A match made in heaven!

Serving size: 4

Cooking Time: 20 Minutes

Ingredients:

- 2 cups broccoli florets, diced
- 1/5 cup button mushroom, diced
- 1 cup firm tofu, cubed
- 2 onions, chopped
- 2 green chilies
- 2 tbsp butter
- 2 tbsp soy sauce
- Salt and pepper to taste
- 1 tsp sugar
- 4 garlic cloves, sliced

Instructions:

In a wok, melt the butter and toss the garlic until they are golden.

Add the onion and toss for 1 minute.

Add the tofu and toss until it becomes golden.

Add the broccoli and mushroom.

Add the soy sauce, green chilies, and salt and pepper.

Cook for about 8 minutes.

Add the sugar. Then, cook for 2 minutes.

Serve hot.

Grilled Salmon Fillets

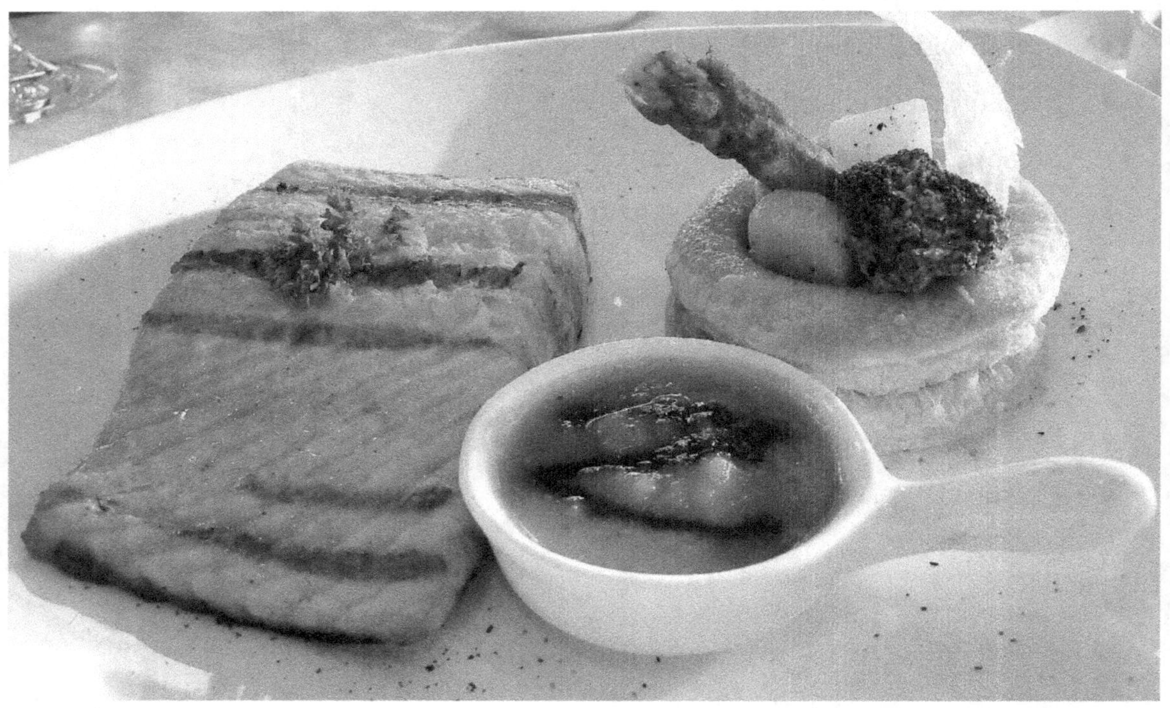

I bet you love salmon, and you want to have it more often for the health benefit it carries. With a recipe like this one, it becomes very easy and quick to include salmon in your everyday menu.

Serving size: 4

Cooking Time: 15 Minutes

Ingredients:

- 4 salmon fillets
- 1 tsp parsley, chopped
- 1 tsp rosemary, chopped
- 1 tsp thyme, chopped
- 2 tbsp lemon juice
- 2 tbsp honey
- Salt and pepper to taste
- 2 tbsp olive oil

Instructions:

Debone the salmon fillets.

Combine the herbs, with honey, lemon juice, and salt and pepper.

Mix well and coat the fillets in it.

In a grilling pan, add the olive oil.

Grill the fish fillets for 2 minutes on each side.

Serve warm.

Deep-Fried Small Fish with Green Beans and Potatoes

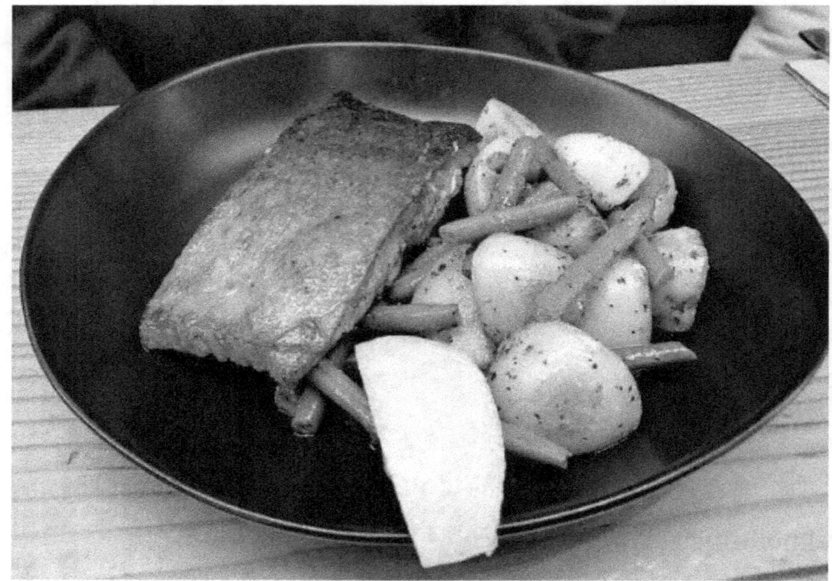

Big fishes do taste good but do you know you can enjoy a good meal with small fishes too? You just have to know how to cook it and what you should combine it with! Here I have fried the small fish and served it with butter tossed potatoes and green beans.

Serving size: 4

Cooking Time: 15 Minutes

Ingredients:

- 4 small fish
- 1 cup green beans, cut in half
- 1 cup potatoes, cut into wedges
- Salt and pepper to taste
- 2 tbsp oil
- 2 tbsp butter
- 2 tbsp chopped chives
- ¼ tsp garlic powder
- 1 tsp paprika
- 1 tsp cumin
- 1 tbsp chopped parsley
- 1 tsp chopped rosemary

Instructions:

Clean the fishes properly. Coat the fish with garlic, salt, paprika, rosemary and cumin.

Let it sit for 10 minutes. In a pan, add the oil.

Fry the fish for 4 minutes from both sides.

Transfer to a serving plate.

In another pan, melt the butter. Add the potatoes.

Add salt, pepper and chives, and toss for 10 minutes.

Transfer to the serving plate.

In the same pan, add the green beans. Add salt, pepper and parsley.

Cook for 4 minutes. Serve with the fish and potatoes.

Lentil Minced Chicken and celery Salad

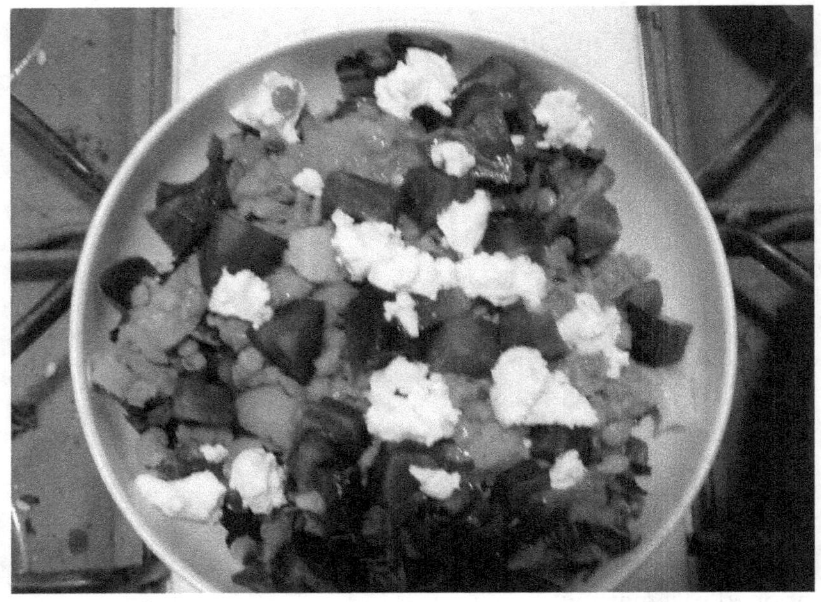

Have you ever tried lentil with celery and minced chicken? The combination would actually surprise you, in a good way!

Serving size: 4

Cooking Time: 15 Minutes

Ingredients:

- 1.5 cups boiled red lentils
- 1.5 cups celery, chopped
- 1.5 cups chicken, minced
- Salt and pepper to taste
- 1 tsp paprika
- 1 tbsp oil
- 1 onion, chopped
- 4 garlic cloves, minced
- 1 tsp dried oregano
- 1 cup torn collard leaves
- 1 tbsp lemon juice

Instructions:

In a large wok, heat the oil. Add the garlic and the onion.

Cook for 2 minutes. Add the minced chicken.

Cook until it gets brown.

Add the boiled lentil and the celery.

Add the oregano, paprika, and salt and pepper.

Cook for 5 minutes. Add the lemon juice and mix well.

Arrange the collard leaves on a serving plate.

Add the chicken mix on top. Serve hot.

Cauliflower Egg Curry

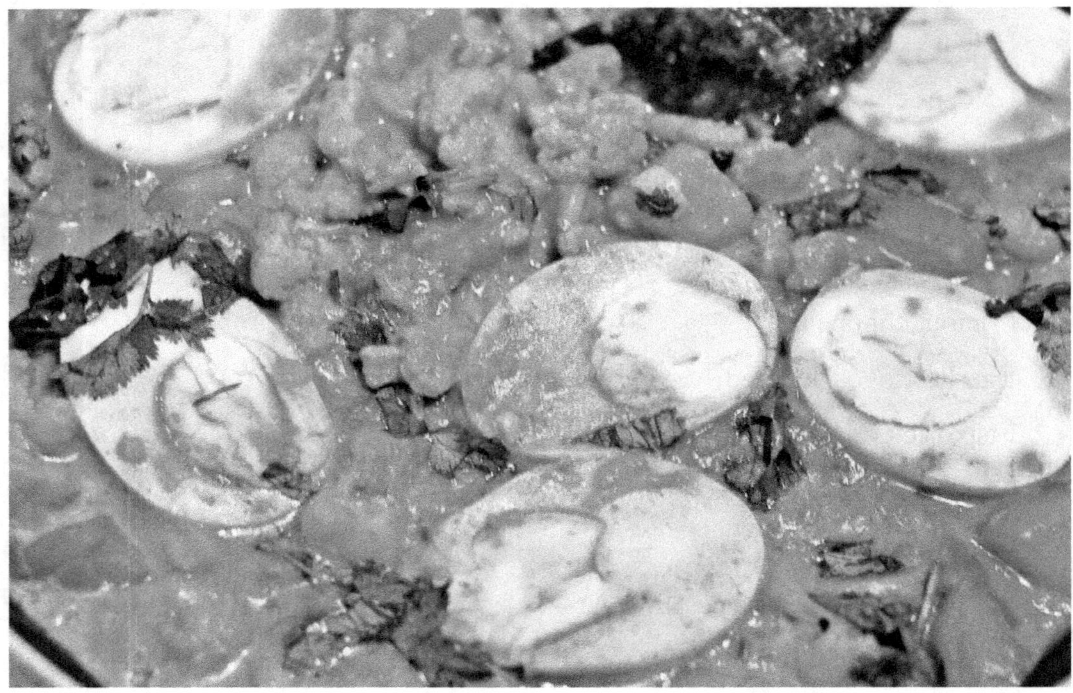

If you have not tried boiled egg curry with cauliflower, then it is time you should try it. They complement each other quite well.

Serving size: 4

Cooking Time: 25 Minutes

Ingredients:

- 4 eggs
- 2 cups cauliflower florets
- Salt and pepper to taste
- 2 green chilies
- 2 tbsp chives, chopped
- 1 tsp parsley, chopped
- 2 white onions, sliced
- ¼ tsp turmeric
- 1 tsp red chili powder
- 1 tsp cumin
- 2 tbsp oil
- 1 tsp ginger paste
- 1 tsp garlic paste
- 1 cup vegetable stock

Instructions:

Hard boil the egg in water for 8 minutes.

Let it cool down and remove the egg shells.

In your pan, heat the oil and fry the eggs until they become golden. Transfer them onto a plate.

Next, in the same pan, add the onion and cook for 1 minute.

Add the ginger and garlic paste. Toss for 1 minute.

Add the turmeric, red chili powder, cumin, salt, pepper and vegetable stock.

Bring it to boil and simmer for 5 minutes.

Add the cauliflower florets and chives. Cook for 5 minutes.

Add the green chilies, parsley and eggs, and cook for 5 minutes.

Serve hot.

Conclusion

Eating clean and grain free is very praiseworthy; because it can reduce weight, help you combat many health issues, and, most importantly, it promotes your controlling eating choice. Half the times our food controls us. The reason you should choose to be grain free is the desire to be fit and active. Being healthy is the ultimate goal. When you eat good food, you invariably feel good about yourself too. On the contrary, when you eat rubbish junk food, you feel very low and lethargic. We all are given only one life, in this short period of time it is only obvious that you should not waste it with food, rather you should make a wise food choice and be productive and happy.

About the Author

Born in New Germantown, Pennsylvania, Stephanie Sharp received a Masters degree from Penn State in English Literature. Driven by her passion to create culinary masterpieces, she applied and was accepted to The International Culinary School of the Art Institute where she excelled in French cuisine. She has married her cooking skills with an aptitude for business by opening her own small cooking school where she teaches students of all ages.

Stephanie's talents extend to being an author as well and she has written over 400 e-books on the art of cooking and baking that include her most popular recipes.

Sharp has been fortunate enough to raise a family near her hometown in Pennsylvania where she, her husband and children live in a beautiful rustic house on an extensive piece of land. Her other passion is taking care of the furry members of her family which include 3 cats, 2 dogs and a potbelly pig named Wilbur.

Watch for more amazing books by Stephanie Sharp coming out in the next few months.

Author's Afterthoughts

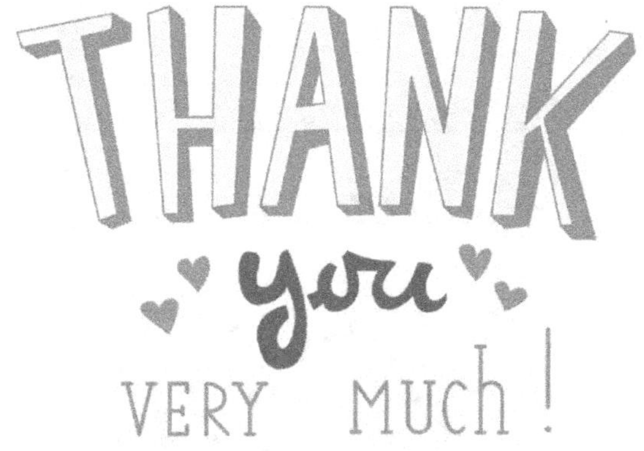

I am truly grateful to you for taking the time to read my book. I cherish all of my readers! Thanks ever so much to each of my cherished readers for investing the time to read this book!

With so many options available to you, your choice to buy my book is an honour, so my heartfelt thanks at reading it from beginning to end!

I value your feedback, so please take a moment to submit an honest and open review on Amazon so I can get valuable insight into my readers' opinions and others can benefit from your experience.

Thank you for taking the time to review!

Stephanie Sharp

For announcements about new releases, please follow my author page on Amazon.com!

You can find that at:

https://www.amazon.com/author/stephanie-sharp

*or Scan **QR-code** below.*